Metabolic Detox: 3 Day Step– By-Step Juice Detox With Recipes

Disclaimer and Terms of Use: Effort has been made to ensure that the information in this book is accurate and complete, however, the author and the publisher do not warrant the accuracy of the information, text and graphics contained within the book due to the rapidly changing nature of science, research, known and unknown facts and internet. The Author and the publisher do not hold any responsibility for errors, omissions or contrary interpretation of the subject matter herein. This book is presented solely for motivational and informational purposes only.

Table of Contents

Introduction

Our body has a natural detoxification and excretory system which helps to eliminate the waste from our body. But, due to the changes in our life style and due to the changes in our food habits, sometimes our body cannot do detoxification effectively. Moreover, the environmental pollution and the use of insecticides and pesticides are making the air we breathe, the food we eat and the water we drink a source to toxic substances. The lifestyle that includes partying and consumption of junk foods and fast foods and alcohol consumption adds to the problem. All these exposures to various toxic items increase the chances of degenerative diseases. Heart diseases, cancer, obesity, high blood pressure and diabetes, gastrointestinal problems are becoming common even in people of young age. The liver is the major detoxifying organ in our body. Our intestine, kidneys and skin also play an important role in the elimination of wastes and toxins from our body. Hence, it is necessary to cleanse and detoxify the whole body at regular intervals. Detoxification is the effective way to remove the toxins from your body and to have a more healthy and energetic body with the help of diet. Here, you are going to get all the necessary information regarding detoxification using juices.

Detoxification Using Juice

When you are opting for detoxification with juices, you are providing the necessary nutrients, minerals, antioxidants, fibers, water, etc. through the juice diet for a few days. When you are detoxifying using juices, you are reducing the stress on the digestive system for a few days and this helps the system to rejuvenate and work with more efficiency after the detoxification. The juices can provide the necessary electrolytes, soluble fibers and trace minerals necessary for the balanced working of our body. During juice detox you will be consuming juices made of raw fruits and vegetables and water for three days. This is considered as one of the fastest method to achieve detoxification as you will not be eating any solid food and the food intake is very low. It is better to consult a doctor before starting a juice diet if you have any pre-existing health problems or if you are doing the detox for more than three days. You can try detoxifying your body using juices prior to making changes in lifestyle or before starting your weight loss program.

The Benefits Of Juice Detoxification

Drinking fresh fruit and vegetables for detoxification has many health benefits.

- You will get the vitamins and minerals from the fresh fruits and vegetables that do not usually consume

- The nutrients are in easily absorbable form to the body as the nutrients get dissolved in the water content

- It helps in improving the digestive ability of your gastrointestinal tract and prevents the problems of the digestive tract

- It cleanses your system and hence you will feel more energetic

- You will get clear and refreshed skin

- Your concentration ability will improve

- You will get good sleep

- The above benefits help your body prevent cardiovascular diseases, cancer, rheumatoid arthritis and various other inflammatory diseases

- The anti-oxidants prevent the oxidative cell damages

- Reduces the harmful effects of pollution on your body

Things To Remember While Detoxifying

You have to consider certain things before you opt for the 3 day juice detoxification.

- You can do this detoxification once in every month. You may feel the hunger pangs and tiredness on the first day, but your body will get adjusted to it in the coming days.

- Always wash and clean the fruits and vegetables before juicing them.

- Clean the juicer properly after each use.

- It is better to prepare fresh juice every time.

- Drink the juices slowly to optimize the absorption of nutrients.

- Go for 30 minutes walk every day.

- Pregnant women should avoid this detoxification.

- Continue to take your regular medication during the detox.

- One or two juices for a day should include green leafy based vegetables.

- If the detox method does not suit you, immediately stop the process.

- Slowly get back to your normal diet after detoxification, do not over eat and introduce foods like grains, meat, and milk one at a time.

Foods To Avoid While Detoxifying

When you are on a fruit and veg. juice detoxification you need to avoid certain foods which affect the effectiveness of the detoxification in a negative way. These foods include

- Red meat, chicken, turkey and other processed meat such as sausages.

- Dairy products such as milk, cream, butter and cheese

- Eggs, potato chips, salted nuts

- Tea, coffee, alcohol and aerated and non-aerated drinks

- Sugar, chocolates and sweets

- Preserved salad dressings

Avoiding these food items helps to detoxify the body faster and to achieve a healthy lifestyle thereafter.

Preparing Yourself For The 3 Day Juice Detox

You may be following the 3 day juice detox plan to cleanse your body or to keep your weight in control. This plan can be easily followed even by the beginners. You can achieve all your cleansing and weight reduction goals with this plan, provided you prepare yourself for the juice detox plan. Though it is not necessary to follow the instruction word by word, it is necessary to understand the basic things and follow the advices to get maximum result. Follow these steps to achieve the most excellent result.

Step- 1

Remove all the food items which are tempting from your refrigerator and kitchen. Fill your refrigerator and kitchen with more healthy fruits and vegetables. Keep the recipes for the juices ready before stating the detoxification

Step-2

Start avoiding meat, fish and eggs one or two days before starting the juice detoxification. This will help the body to adjust to the detox plan more easily. You can also start avoiding sugar and fats before starting the detox. This will give better and faster results, especially if you want to cleanse as well as losing weight.

Step -3

Do not follow the plan as such. You can make necessary changes according to your fruit and veg. preferences. You can experiment with your favorite veggies and fruits.

Step- 4

Do not include any solid foods other than fruits and vegetables during this 3 day body cleansing plan. This will overthrow your effort to cleanse and detox the body.   You can use any type of juice for three days.

Step-5

It is normal for people to feel headaches and cravings for food when they are on the detox. You can try having some extra juice to control the craving. It will be difficult to focus on the juice diet first day, but try to stay on the juice.

Step-6

It is necessary that you drink plenty of water when you are on a juice diet. Drink at least 16oz of water after taking your juices. The water helps to eliminate the toxic substances from the body effectively. It also maintains the acidic balance of the body.

Step- 7

Always start your day with the juice of ½ lemon mixed with 16 ounces warm water. This will help to cleanse the digestive system and helps in better digestion of the food you are consuming afterwards.

Step -8

To get the best results and to avoid the cravings for food it is better to have 4-6 juices per day. Each time you can consume 16-20 ounces of juice. You can add natural spices and flavors of your choice but avoid the use of salt. The final juice of the day should be taken at least 3 hours before hitting the bed.

How To Make Juice Detox More Effective?

You can make the juice detox more effective by following certain simple things

Mild Physical Activity

You should cut down your rigorous fitness exercises during the detox days. However, it is necessary to continue mild physical activities like walking or cycling at moderate speed. This will improve the circulation of blood and lymphatic fluids in the body, helping in easy elimination of wastes.

Promoting Elimination Of Toxins

The toxins which are mobilized during the detox plan should get eliminated from the body or they will get reabsorbed into the body system. You can try enema or herbal laxatives to promote the elimination of wastes.

Reducing Stress

Stress will have a negative effect on health and it also affects the effectiveness of detoxification plan. Keep your mind and body calm by meditation, mild yoga practices or by relaxation of the body by massages.

The 3 - Day Cleanse Recipes

Once you are through with all the important steps that you need to take to start the three day body detox program in your bid to lose weight and to stay fit and healthy, you are all set to learn about the recipes that you need to prepare for these three days. It is also important for you to continue to start your day with lime juice prepared in hot water and with a dash of ginger. You should also make sure that you end your day with a cup of hot herbal tea.

On all the three days of your juice fasting plan you will need to take a total of five juices every day and must also eat a meal that consists of fresh and organic vegetables and fruits in order to enjoy the maximum benefits of the cleanse program. You also need to make sure that you eat the fresh fruits and vegetables as your dinner and at the end of the day as this will help you to feel full. You will not be falling prey to stomach cravings or getting the feeling of starving at night. In fact, you can also get a good night's sleep if you do not have the feeling of starving or deprivation.

You will be able to reap the maximum benefits of juice fasting by following the following five juice diet for a three day weekend so that you get your entire system to be cleansed off from the toxins and other wastes. You will feel lighter and healthier by the end of this 3-day weekend cleanse program.

The following are the recipes that you must take every day for the 3 day weekend cleanse program and you need to take the right juices at the right times all the 3 days to get the best benefits.

1. Breakfast: Ginger Apple And Carrot Juice

The first juice for breakfast will be the carrot and apple juice and make sure to note the time when you are having your breakfast juice on the first day. Try to consume this breakfast juice on the 2nd and 3rd day of your weekend juice fast plan at just about the same time. The ingredients that you will need are:

Ingredients Needed

- 3 carrots
- 2 apples
- One inch piece of ginger

Preparation

➢ Cut the carrots into medium sized cubes and put it in a blender.

- ➤ Add the cut apples as well in the blender.

- ➤ Now add one inch piece of fresh ginger and then blend all these three ingredients on high to make a smoothie.

- ➤ Strain the contents from a blender into a glass that is filled with ice cubes on the bottom.

- ➤ Drink and enjoy your breakfast.

- ➤ If you need some more extra sweetness to your breakfast, then you can add a tablespoon of honey in the blender along with other ingredients.

2. Mid Morning Juice: Mean Lean Green Juice

It is very important for you to take a mid morning juice every day for the three days of your cleanse plan as you are only on a liquid diet and the body will need a lot of vitamins, minerals and other important ingredients to function properly. The mid morning juice can be taken after a couple of hours of having your breakfast detox juice. Make sure that you take the mid morning juice on all three days more or less at the same time to get good results.

Ingredients Needed

- 2 apples

- 4 celery stalks

- ½ piece lemon

- 1 cucumber

- 6 to 8 kale leaves

- 1 inch ginger

Preparation

- ➤ Remove the skin of the cucumber and cut the cucumber into small, medium sized pieces so that it can easily blend in the blender.

- ➤ After adding the cucumber pieces into the blender, now add cut pieces of two apples and the kale leaves.

- ➤ Now squeeze ½ piece of lemon juice into the blender and add an inch of ginger piece along with the celery stalks.

- ➤ Blend all these ingredients thoroughly in a blender on high speed for about 2 minutes.

- ➤ Now, strain the contents of the blender into a vessel.

> Fill a tall juice glass with 2/3rd of ice cubes or crushed ice and then pour the special green juice into the glass.

> Drink it immediately.

3. Gazpacho Juice For Lunch

The third juice that you will be taking on the first day of your three day juice fast plan is the Gazpacho juice which will be your lunch juice. It is a very healthy juice that has all minerals, vitamins, proteins and antioxidants needed to keep your body healthy. You can have your lunch juice after two hours of having your mid morning juice. Make sure that you take the lunch juice on all the three days of your juice detox plan at the same time.

Ingredients

- 4 ripe and plum tomatoes

- 1 small red onion

- 2 cups parsley, include both leaves and stem and they should be roughly chopped

- 1 large cucumber, de-skinned and cut into small pieces

- 1 red bell pepper

- Juice of one lime

- 2 celery stalks

Preparation

➢ Take a blender and add the cut piece of cucumber and 2 cups of chopped parsley and blend it for 30 seconds.

➢ Now, add the tomatoes and celery and then blend for another 30 seconds.

➢ Next, you got to add a small red onion, red bell pepper and the lime juice into the blended mixture.

➢ Now blend for 2 minutes on high until all ingredients get mixed and turns into a paste form.

➢ Strain the contents of the blender in a vessel.

➢ Now take a tall glass and fill half the juice glass with ice. Pour the strained juice into the tall glass and drink it immediately.

4. Afternoon Juice: Green And Citrus Mix Juice

The fourth juice of the day will be the afternoon juice that you need to take for three days in the afternoon during the 3 day detox juice fast plan. This is a juice that contains greens and citrus as its main ingredients. You need to take this afternoon juice after two and a half to three hours of having your lunch juice. Make it a point to drink the afternoon juice at the same time on all the three days to enjoy good detoxification results at the end of the program.

Ingredients

- 1 medium sized cucumber

- Swiss chard leaves (8)

- 6 Clementine

- Kale leaves (6 to 8)

Preparation

➢ Peel off the skin of the cucumber and cut it into medium sized pieces and then add it in a blender.

➢ Now to this add Clementine, Swiss chard and kale leaves. Add a few drops of lime juice to add more citrus taste.

- ➢ Blend all these ingredients till they become a smooth fine paste.

- ➢ Strain the contents of the blender into a vessel.

- ➢ Now, take a glass that is three-fourths filled with crushed ice and pour the strained juice into the tall glass.

- ➢ Drink it immediately.

5. Pre- Dinner Juice: Sunset Blend Juice

The last juice of the day is the pre-dinner juice that you need to take after three hours of having your afternoon special juice. It is important for you to drink this pre-dinner juice exactly at the same time on all the three days of your juice fast plan program. As this is the last juice of the day, enjoy it to the fullest.

Ingredients

- A medium sized carrot

- A large sweet potato

- A couple of delicious and ripe red apples

- 2 big red beets

- 1 red bell pepper

- An orange (optional)

Preparation

➢ Cut the medium sized carrot, sweet potato and the large beets into cubes so that they can be easily blended in the blender or food processor.

➢ Now add all these three ingredients into the blender and blend it for a minute.

➢ After this you add coarsely cut red apples, orange and red bell pepper in the mixture and blend again for two minutes or until the ingredients inside trunks smooth.

➢ Now strain the special sunset blend juice into a clean vessel.

➢ Fill ½ the tall juice glass with ice cubes and then pour the juice into the glass.

➢ Drink it immediately.

6. Dinner Recipes

After you have completed taking in all the five juices for the day, you now have a chance to eat something solid for dinner. You can take your dinner about one and a half hours after you have taken your last juice, which is the pre-dinner juice. The following are some of the dinner meal recipes that you can choose from to complete your detox plan for the day.

a) Sweet Potato And Carrot Healthy Fries

You can choose to go for this dish as your dinner when you are on a three day juice detox plan. The main reason why you need to take dinner at night during the detox plan is because you do not want to feel hungry in the odd hours at night and you can get a good and peaceful sleep with the feeling that your stomach is full. In fact, the vegetables will give you a feeling that your stomach is full.

Ingredients

- 2 large carrots
- 2 medium sized sweet potatoes
- ½ tsp sea salt
- 2 tbsp olive oil
- ¼ tsp pepper
- ½ tsp freshly ground cumin powder

Preparation

- You need to preheat your oven at 425ºF before starting the cooking process.

- Peel the skin of the sweet potatoes and carrots. Cut potatoes into half slices lengthwise and then cut each of the slices into four wedges.

- Cut the carrots crosswise into two halves. Now, slice each of the half lengthwise to get two long pieces and then cut each of these pieces into 2 to 3 wedges.

- Make sure that the size of the potatoes and the carrot wedges are more or less the same.

- Now put the potato and carrot wedges into a bowl and toss the pieces with cumin powder, pepper and salt.

- Arrange the tossed vegetables on a baking tray and bake it in the preheated oven for 30 minutes.

- Make sure that the flesh of the carrot and potatoes are tender and the outside of the wedges get browned so that you get a crispy feeling when you bite the wedges.

➢ You will enjoy this new dinner meal with aromatic cumin spice and olive oil dressing.

b) Avocado And Kale Salad

The avocado and kale salad is the perfect dinner that you need after a five time detox juice diet. It is a salad that is very easy o make and make sure that you only consume the salad just one and hours after having the last pre-dinner juice. Another thing to note is that you need to have your dinner at the right time on all the three days of your juice fasting plan.

Ingredients

- ½ avocado that is diced

- 1 handful of red cabbage that is coarsely chopped

- 1 finely chopped tomato

- 4 handfuls of kale

- ½ cup olive oil

- 1 tbsp honey

- ¼ cup fresh basil or ½ tsp dried basil

- 4 finely chopped garlic cloves

- ¼ teaspoon coarsely ground black pepper

- 1 tbsp balsamic vinegar

- Sea salt to taste

Procedure

> You need to chop the kale leaves and also chop red cabbage, avocado and tomato.

> Mix all these ingredients in a bowl.

> You need to mix the dressing in a separate bowl.

> The dressing includes olive oil, balsamic vinegar, sea salt, garlic, black pepper and honey. Mix them well.

> You will just need one or two tablespoons of this dressing for your recipe. You can save the remaining dressing and use it when making other salads.

> You need to store the cut vegetables in the refrigerator and only dress it with olive oil mixture when you are ready to have your dinner.

➢ Once prepared, you are ready to binge into it. You are sure to enjoy a solid dinner after just having healthy juices for the whole day.

www.ingramcontent.com/pod-product-compliance
Lightning Source LLC
Chambersburg PA
CBHW061949280526
45787CB00004B/1790